The New
Keto Chaffle
Recipes

The Ultimate Waffle Recipes to Lose Weight, Stay
Healthy, and Maintain Your Ketogenic Diet

Caroline Betram

the reader will render any resulting actions solely under their purview. There are no scenarios in which the publisher or the original author of this work can be in any fashion deemed liable for any hardship or damages that may befall them after undertaking information described herein.

Additionally, the information in the following pages is intended only for informational purposes and should thus be thought of as universal. As befitting its nature, it is presented without assurance regarding its prolonged validity or interim quality. Trademarks that are mentioned are done without written consent and can in no way be considered an endorsement from the trademark holder.

Table of Contents

INTRODUCTION

The name "Chaffles" comes from the union of cheese + waffles, just because it is the cheese the main ingredient for their realization, along with eggs and all the various types of condiments you can use.

The combinations can be endless. It is precisely the substitution of flour for cheese that makes chaffles low in carbohydrates. Besides, the egg's addition increases the fat intake-ideal for those following the ketogenic diet.

Chaffles is the most recent famous nourishment in the keto world. This straightforward keto formula is fresh, brilliant dark-colored, sans sugar, low-carb, and exceptionally simple to make.

Chaffles are turning into somewhat of a furor with supporters of the keto diet. They're less fastidious to make than most keto bread recipes and they're anything but difficult to customize. You can transform the fundamental formula for a chaffle into your creation, running from flavorful to sweet and anything in the middle. You can likewise change the sort of cheddar you use, delivering significant changes in the flavor and surface of the chaffle.

You can enjoy this mouth-watering dish in every meal of your day, there are countless combinations of low-carb ketogenic ingredients available, so it's easy to find a chaffle one to love!

Depending on how you serve them, they can be delicious sweet desserts, nutrient breakfast food, or a quick snack, try them in a sandwich, pizza, and French toast variations!

The best option to make them is the Chaffle Maker, but you can prepare yourself one with a regular Waffle maker or even a nonstick saucepan.

Some people does not like the taste that comes from the egg as base ingredients, here some tips on how to avoid too much eggy taste:

- *Increase the sugar quantity.*
- *Add milk powder.*
- *Add lime, lemon, or orange juice. Use a teaspoon of juice per 3 eggs.*
- *Add some rind. Use a quarter teaspoon per 3 eggs.*
- *Let chaffle cool completely.*
- *Use egg whites instead of whole eggs.*

To reheat the chaffles, pop them into the waffle maker or oven, or toaster for few minutes.

You can store cooked chaffles in the freezer for up to three months. You can also store cooked chaffles for up to three days at room temperature or one week in the refrigerator.

Keto Chaffle Recipes

CHOCOLATE CHAFFLE

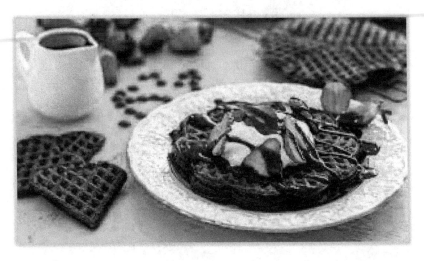

5 minutes

5 minutes

1 Servings

INGREDIENTS

2 tablespoons of coconut flour

1 tablespoon of cocoa powder

1 egg, beaten

1 ounce cream cheese, soft

1 teaspoon of vanilla extract

1 tablespoon of stevia

DIRECTIONS

1. In a bowl mix the flour with cocoa, egg and other ingredients and beat well.

2. Preheat the waffle iron to medium-high heat, pour the chaffle mixture into it, close the waffle iron, cook for 5 minutes, transfer to a plate and serve.

ALMOND FLOUR CHAFFLE WITH MOZZARELLA

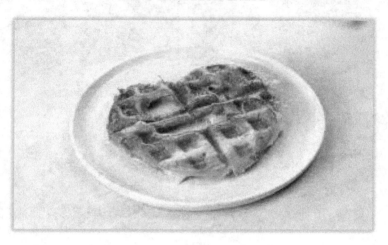

5 minutes

8 minutes

2 Servings

INGREDIENTS

1 large egg, beaten

½ cup of mozzarella cheese, shredded

2 tbsp almond flour

¼ tsp baking powder

DIRECTIONS

1. Heat up the mini waffle maker.

2. Add all the ingredients to a small mixing bowl and combine well.

3. Pour half of the batter into the waffle maker and cook for 4 minutes until brown. Repeat with the rest of the batter to make another chaffle.

4. Let cool for 3 minutes to let chaffles get crispy. Serve and enjoy!

PESTO CHAFFLE

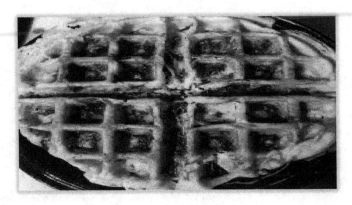

10 minutes

13 minutes

2 Servings

INGREDIENTS

1 egg

½ cup shredded cheddar cheese

For topping:

2 tbsp marinara sauce

2 tbsp mozzarella cheese, shredded

1 tbsp olives, minced

1 tomato, sliced

1 tbsp keto pesto sauce

DIRECTIONS

1. Heat up the waffle maker and preheat oven at 400°.

2. Add egg and shredded cheese to a small mixing bowl and combine well.

3. Pour half of the batter into the waffle maker and cook for 4 minutes until golden brown. Repeat with the rest of the batter to make another chaffle.

4. Let cool for 3 minutes to let chaffles get crispy.

5. Spread the marinara sauce and the keto pesto on the chaffle.

6. Top with olives, mozzarella cheese and olives.

7. Bake the chaffles for approx. 5 minutes.

11

CREAM CHEESE CHAFFLE

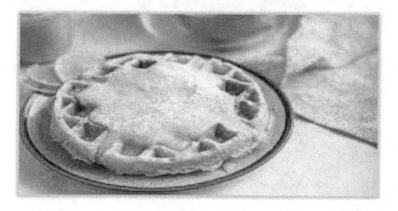

5 minutes

8 minutes

2 Servings

INGREDIENTS

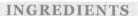

1 egg, beaten

1 oz. cream cheese

½ teaspoon vanilla

4 teaspoons sweetener

¼ teaspoon baking powder Cream cheese

DIRECTIONS

1. Preheat now your waffle maker.

2. Add all the ingredients in a bowl.

3. Mix well.

4. Pour half of the batter into your waffle maker.

5. Seal the device.

6. Cook for 4 minutes.

7. Remove now the chaffle from your waffle maker.

8. Make the second one using the same steps.

9. Spread remaining cream cheese on top before serving.

BANANA NUT CHAFFLE

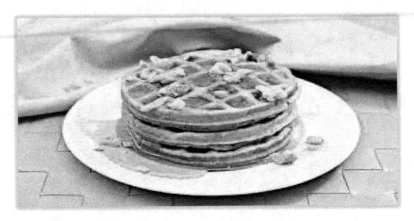

10 minutes

10 minutes

2 Servings

INGREDIENTS

1 egg

1 tablespoon cream cheese, softened, room temperature

Keto So 1 tbs. Sugar-Free Cheesecake Pudding

Optional Ingredient

1/2 cup mozzarella cheese

1 tbs. fruit sauce

1/4 teaspoon of vanilla extract

1/4 teaspoon banana extract

DIRECTIONS

1. Prehat mini chaffle maker.

2. Put the eggs in an average bowl and add all other ingredients to the egg mixture and blend until thoroughly mixed.

3. Add half the butter and mix, then cook for around 5 minutes until mixture is golden.

4. Remove the finished chaffle and add another portion of the mixture to cook another chaffle.

5. Serve with your favorite toppings and enjoy it hot.

LIME PIE CHAFFLE

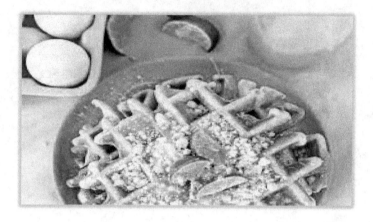

5 minutes

4 minutes

1 Servings

INGREDIENTS

1 egg

1/4 cup Almond flour

2 teaspoons cream cheese

1 teaspoon powdered sweetener Swerve or Monk Fruit

½ teaspoon lime extract or 1 teaspoon freshly squeezed lime juice

½ teaspoon baking powder

½ teaspoon lime zest

Pinch of salt

DIRECTIONS

1. Preheat the waffle maker.

2. Add all chaffle ingredients into the blender and blend at high speed until smooth and creamy. Pour mixture into the waffle maker.

3. Cook for four minutes maximum until golden brown.

4. Make the frosting: mix all ingredients for frosting and combine well.

5. Let cool the chaffle and serve!

Cream Cheese Lime Frosting:

4 ounces cream cheese softened

4 tablespoons butter

2 teaspoons powdered sweetener Swerve or Monk Fruit

1 teaspoon lime extract

½ teaspoon lime zest

KETO SMORES CHAFFLE

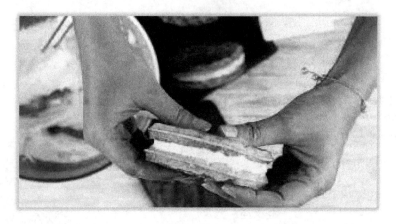

10 minutes

20 minutes

3 Servings

INGREDIENTS

1 large Egg

½ c. Mozzarella cheese shredded

½ tsp Vanilla extract

2 tbs Swerve brown

½ tbs Psyllium Husk Powder optional

¼ tsp Baking Powder

Pinch of pink salt

¼ Lily's Original Dark Chocolate Bar

2 tbs Keto Marshmallow Creme Fluff Recipe

DIRECTIONS

1. Make the batch of Keto Marshmallow Creme Fluff.

2. Whisk the egg until creamy.

3. Add vanilla and Swerve Brown, mix well.

4. Mix in the shredded cheese and blend.

5. Then add Psyllium Husk Powder, baking powder and salt.

6. Mix until well incorporated, let the batter rest 3-4 minutes.

7. Prep/plug in your waffle maker to preheat.

8. Spread ½ batter on the waffle maker and cook 3-4 minutes.

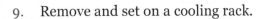

9. Remove and set on a cooling rack.

10. Cook second half of batter same, then remove to cool.

11. Once cool, assemble the chaffles with the marshmallow fluff and chocolate:

12. Using 2 tbs marshmallow and ¼ bar of Lily's Chocolate.

13. Eat as is, or toast for a melty and gooey Smore sandwich!

RASPBERRIES CHAFFLES

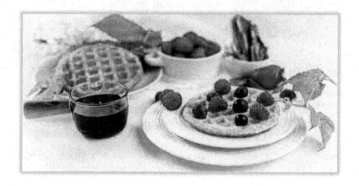

5 minutes

5 minutes

2 Servings

INGREDIENTS

1 egg

1/2 cup mozzarella cheese, shredded

1 tbsp. almond flour

1/4 cup raspberry puree

1 tbsp. coconut flour for topping

DIRECTIONS

1. Preheat your waffle maker in line with the manufacturer's instructions.

2. Grease your waffle maker with cooking spray.

3. Mix together egg, almond flour, and raspberry purée.

4. Add cheese and mix until well combined.

5. Pour batter into the waffle maker.

6. Close the lid.

7. Cook for about 3-4 minutes Utes or until waffles are cooked and not soggy.

8. Once cooked, remove from the maker.

9. Sprinkle coconut flour on top and enjoy!

COCONUT CHAFFLE

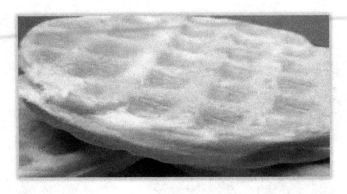

5 minutes

10 minutes

4 Servings

INGREDIENTS

½ cup of cream cheese, soft

spoon of coconut pulp, unsweetened and chopped

teaspoons of coconut oil, dissolved

1 tablespoon of coconut flour

3 eggs, beaten

1 tablespoon of erythritol

1 teaspoon of vanilla extract

½ teaspoon of almond extract

DIRECTIONS

1. In a bowl, combine the cream cheese with the melted coconut oil and other ingredients and blend well.

2. Heat the waffle iron over high heat, pour in ¼ of the batter, close the waffle maker, cook for 10 minutes and transfer to a plate.

3. Repeat with the rest of the batter and serve the chaffles hot.

KETO SWEET BREAD CHAFFLE

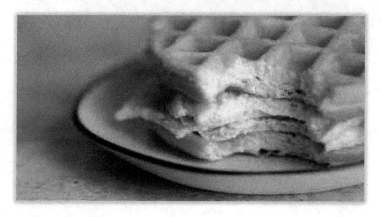

10 minutes

3 minutes

1 Servings

INGREDIENTS

1 tbs almond flour

1 egg

1 tbs mayo we love this brand of mayo

1/8 tsp baking powder

1 tbs Allulose sweetener powdered

1/4 tsp cinnamon

1/8 tsp salt

DIRECTIONS

1. Stir all ingredients: together. Let rest for 5 min.

2. Stir again.

3. Preheat the mini waffle iron

4. Put half of dough in mini waffle maker.

5. Cook 3 minutes.

6. Repeat. Let cool.

PUMPKIN CHAFFLE WITH MAPLE SYRUP

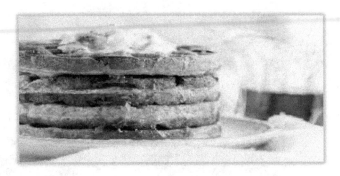

10 minutes

16 minutes

2 Servings

INGREDIENTS

2 eggs, beaten

½ cup Mozzarella cheese, shredded

1 teaspoon coconut flour

¾ teaspoon baking powder

¾ teaspoon pumpkin pie spice

2 teaspoons pureed pumpkin

4 teaspoons heavy whipping cream

½ teaspoon vanilla Pinch salt

2 teaspoons maple syrup (sugar-free)

DIRECTIONS

1. Turn your waffle maker on.

2. Mix all the ingredients except maple syrup in a large bowl.

3. Pour half of the batter into your waffle maker.

4. Close and cooking for minutes.

5. Transfer to a plate to cool for 2 minutes.

6. Repeat the steps with the remaining mixture.

7. Drizzle the maple syrup on top of the chaffles before serving.

CHICKEN JALAPENO POPPER CHAFFLE

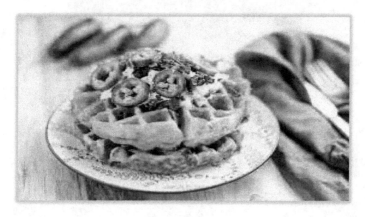

5 minutes

10 minutes

2 Servings

INGREDIENTS

1/2 cup canned chicken breast

1/4 cup cheddar cheese

1/8 cup parmesan cheese

1 egg

1 diced jalapeno (raw or pickled)

1/8 teaspoon onion powder

1/8 teaspoon of garlic powder

1 teaspoon of cream cheese

DIRECTIONS

1. Preheat mini chaffle maker. In an average bowl, add all ingredients and stir together till it's completely blended.

2. Half this mixture and pour a part of the mixture into a mini chaffle maker and cook for a minimum of five minutes.

3. Optional toppings: sour cream, ranch dressing, hot sauce, coriander, leek, feta cheese, jalapeno!

HALLOUMI CHEESE CHAFFLE

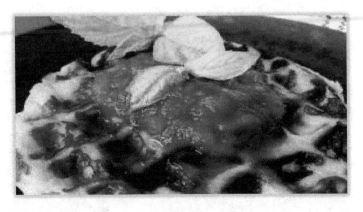

3 minutes

6 minutes

1 Servings

INGREDIENTS

3-ounce Halloumi cheese

2 tablespoons keto Pasta sauce – optional

DIRECTIONS

1. Slice halloumi cheese into half-inch slices.

2. Sprinkle with cheese into the bottom of the waffle maker.

3. Preheat the waffle maker.

4. Cook for three to six minutes until golden brown.

5. Let cool for few minutes.

6. Add keto pasta sauce and serve!

KETO CHAFFLE GARLIC CHEESY BREAD STICKS

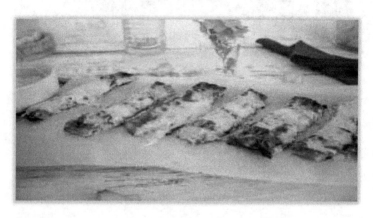

3 minutes

10 minutes

8 Servings

INGREDIENTS

1 medium egg

1/2 cup mozzarella cheese grated

2 tablespoons almond flour

1/2 teaspoon garlic powder

1/2 teaspoon oregano

1/2 teaspoon salt

Topping:

2 tablespoons butter, unsalted softened

DIRECTIONS

1. Turn on your waffle maker and lightly grease it (I give it a light spray with olive oil)

2. In a bowl, beat the egg.

3. Add the mozzarella, almond flour, garlic powder, oregano and salt and mix well.

4. Spoon the batter into your waffle maker (mine is a square double waffle and this mixture covers both waffle sections. If you are using a smaller waffle maker spoon half the mixture in at a time).

5. I spoon my mixture into the centre of my waffle maker and gently spread it out towards the edges.

1/2 teaspoon garlic powder

1/4 cup mozzarella cheese grate

6. Close the lid and cook for 5 minutes.

7. Using tongs, remove the cooked waffles and cut into 4 strips for each waffle.

8. Place the sticks on a tray and pre-heat the grill.

9. Mix the butter with the garlic powder and spread over the sticks.

10. Sprinkle the mozzarella over the sticks and place under the grill for 2-3 minutes until the cheese has melted and bubbling.

11. Eat immediately!

BASIC CHAFFLES RECIPE FOR SANDWICHES

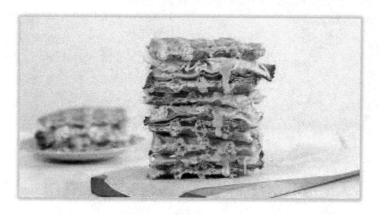

5 minutes

5 minutes

2 Servings

INGREDIENTS

1/2 cup mozzarella cheese, shredded

1 large egg

2 tbsps. Almond flour

1/2 tsp psyllium husk powder

1/4 tsp baking powder

DIRECTIONS

1. Grease your Belgian waffle maker with cooking spray.

2. Beat the egg with a fork; once the egg is beaten, add almond flour, husk powder, and baking powder.

3. Add cheese to the egg mixture and mix until combined.

4. Pour batter in the center of Belgian waffle and close the lid.

5. Cook chaffles for about 2-3 minutes Utes until well cooked.

6. Carefully transfer the chaffles to plate.

7. The chaffles are perfect for a sandwich base.

PUMPKIN AND AVOCADO CHAFFLE

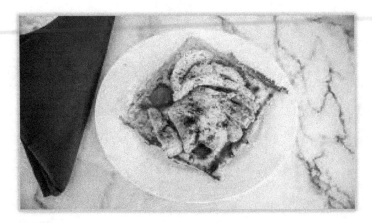

5 minutes

5 minutes

2 Servings

INGREDIENTS

½ cup of cream

1 avocado, peeled, pitted and mashed

1 spoon of coconut flour

2 Eggs, beaten

2 tablespoons of steering

2 and a half tablespoons of pumpkin puree

2 tablespoons of cream cheese, soft

DIRECTIONS

1. In a bowl combine the cream with the avocado, the pumpkin puree and the other ingredients and blend.

2. Heat the waffle iron over high heat, pour in ¼ of the batter, close the waffle maker, cook for 5 minutes and transfer to a plate.

3. Repeat with the rest of the batter and serve the chaffles hot.

EGG-FREE ALMOND FLOUR CHAFFLES

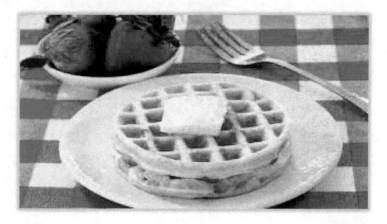

5 minutes

10 minutes

2 Servings

INGREDIENTS

2 tablespoons cream cheese, softened

1 cup mozzarella cheese, shredded

2 tablespoons almond flour

1 teaspoon organic baking powder

DIRECTIONS

1. Preheat a mini waffle iron and then grease it.

2. In a medium bowl, place all ingredients: and with a fork, mix until well combined.

3. Place half of the mixture into preheated waffle iron and cook for about 4-5 minutes or until golden brown.

4. Repeat with the remaining mixture. Serve warm.

VANILLA KETO CHAFFLE

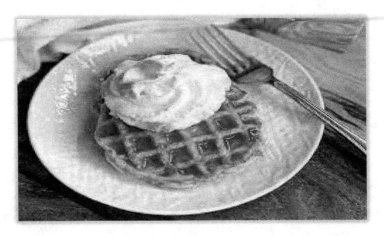

3 minutes

4 minutes

1 Servings

INGREDIENTS

1 egg

1/2 cup cheddar cheese, shredded

1/2 tsp vanilla extract

DIRECTIONS

1. Switch on your waffle maker according to manufacturer's Directions.

2. Crack egg and combine with cheddar cheese in a tiny bowl.

3. Add vanilla extract and combine thoroughly.

4. Place half batter on waffle maker and spread evenly.

5. Cook for 4 minutes or until as desired.

6. Gently Remove now from waffle maker and set aside for 2 minutes so it cools down and become crispy.

7. Repeat for remaining batter.

CARROT CHAFFLE CAKE

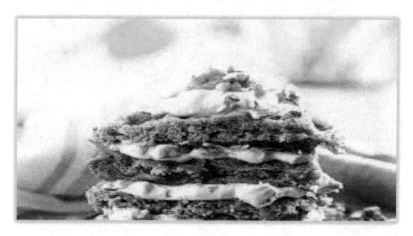

10 minutes

8 minutes

6 Servings

INGREDIENTS

1/2 cup chopped
carrots 1 egg

2 T butter melted

2 T heavy whipped
cream

3/4 cup almond flour

1 walnut chopped

2 T powder sweetener

2 tsp. cinnamon

1 tsp. pumpkin spice

1 tsp. baking powder

**Cream cheese
frosting:**

DIRECTIONS

1. Mix dry ingredients such as almond flour, cinnamon, pumpkin spices, baking powder, powdered sweeteners, and walnut pieces.

2. Add the grated carrots, eggs, melted butter and cream.

3. Add a 3T batter to a preheated mini chaffle maker.

4. Cook for 2 1 / 2-3 minutes.

5. Mix the frosting ingredients with a hand mixer with a whisk until well mixed Stack chaffles and add frosting between each layer!

4 oz cream cheese softened

1/4 cup powdered sweetener

1 teaspoon of vanilla extract

1-2 T heavy whipped cream according to your preferred consistency

KETO BIRTHDAY CAKE CHAFFLE

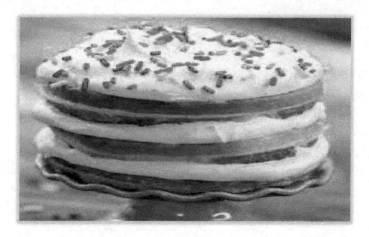

3 minutes

3 minutes

2 Servings

INGREDIENTS

2 eggs

1/4 cup almond flour

1 teaspoon coconut flour

2 tablespoons melted butter

2 tablespoons cream cheese

1 teaspoon cake batter extract

½ teaspoon vanilla extract

½ teaspoon baking powder

DIRECTIONS

1. Preheat the waffle maker.

2. Meanwhile, add all chaffle cake ingredients to the blender and process on high until creamy.

3. Let rest for one minute.

4. Next, add two to three tablespoons of batter to the waffle maker.

5. Cook for two to three minutes.

6. Next, prepare vanilla frosting and whipped cream in another bowl.

7. Add all ingredients for the frosting and combine well until thick.

8. Let cool the chaffle cake and garnish with the whipped cream vanilla frosting.

*2 tablespoons Swerve
confectioners
sweetener or Monk
Fruit*

*1/4 teaspoon Xanthan
powder*

*Whipped Cream
Vanilla Frosting:*

*½ cup heavy
whipping cream*

*2 tablespoons Swerve
confectioners
sweetener or Monk
Fruit*

*½ teaspoon vanilla
extract*

KETO CREAM CHEESE MINI CHAFFLE WAFFLES

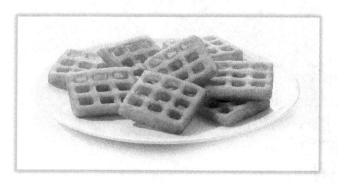

3 minutes

8 minutes

2 Servings

INGREDIENTS

2 tsp Coconut Flour

4 tsp Swerve/Monkfruit

1/4 tsp Baking Powder

1 Whole Egg room temp

1 oz Cream Cheese room temp

1/2 tsp Vanilla Extract

DIRECTIONS

1. Gather all the ingredients. Note - For quick room temperature eggs, submerge egg in warm water for 3-5 min.

2. For quick room temperature cream cheese, take needed amount and microwave for 10-15 sec.

3. Pre-heat waffle iron.

4. In a small mixing bowl, add Coconut Flour, Swerve/Monkfruit, baking powder and mix.

5. Next, add egg, cream cheese, vanilla extract and mix with a whisk until well combined.

6. Pour batter into waffle iron and cook for 3-4 min until browned to liking. Enjoy with your favorite waffle toppings.

KETO COCOA CHAFFLES

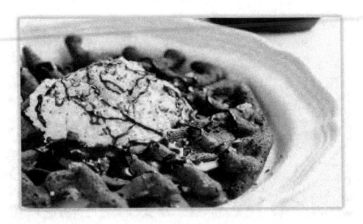

5 minutes

5 minutes

2 Servings

INGREDIENTS

1 large egg

1/2 cup shredded cheddar cheese

1 tbsp. cocoa powder

2 tbsps. almond flour

DIRECTIONS

1. Preheat your round waffle maker on medium-high heat.

2. Mix together egg, cheese, almond flour, cocoa powder and vanilla in a small mixing bowl.

3. Pour chaffles mixture into the center of the waffle iron.

4. Close the waffle maker and let cook for 3-5 minutes Utes or until waffle is golden brown and set.

5. Carefully remove chaffles from the waffle maker.

6. Serve hot and enjoy!

RHUBARB CHAFFLES

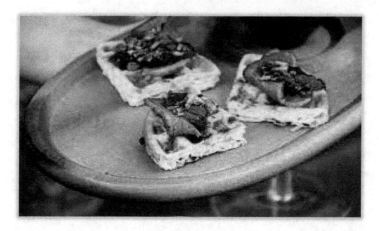

10 minutes

6 minutes

3 Servings

INGREDIENTS

½ cup of rhubarb, chopped

¼ cup of cream

3 tablespoons of cream cheese, soft

2 tablespoons of almond flour

2 beaten eggs

2 tablespoons of steering

½ teaspoon of vanilla extract

½ teaspoon of ground nutmeg

DIRECTIONS

1. In a bowl, mix the rhubarb with the cream, cream cheese and other ingredients and beat well.

2. Heat the waffle iron over high heat, pour in 1/3 of the batter, close the waffle maker, cook for 5 minutes and transfer to a plate.

3. Repeat with the rest of the chaffle batter and serve.

BELGIAN CHAFFLES

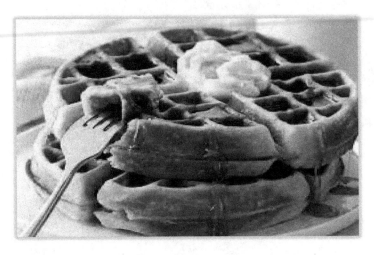

10 minutes

10 minutes

2 Servings

INGREDIENTS

2 eggs

1 cup Reduced-fat Cheddar cheese, shredded

DIRECTIONS

1. Turn on waffle maker to heat and oil it with cooking spray.

2. Whisk eggs in a bowl, add cheese. Stir until well-combined.

3. Pour mixture into waffle maker and cook for 6 minutes until done. Let it cool a little to crisp before serving.

YOGURT CHAFFLES

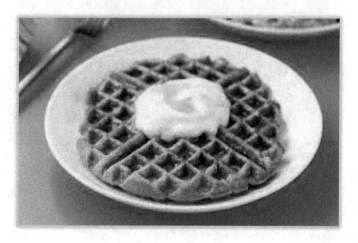

5 minutes

5 minutes

3 Servings

INGREDIENTS

½ cup shredded mozzarella

1 egg

2 Tbsp ground almonds

½ tsp psyllium husk

¼ tsp baking powder

1 Tbsp yogurt

DIRECTIONS

1. Turn on waffle maker to heat and oil it with cooking spray.

2. Whisk eggs in a bowl.

3. Add in remaining ingredients except mozzarella and mix well.

4. Add mozzarella and mix once again. Let it sit for 5 minutes.

5. Add ⅓ cup batter into each waffle mold.

6. Close and cook for 4-5 minutes.

7. Repeat now with remaining batter.

SWEET ZUCCHINI CHAFFLE

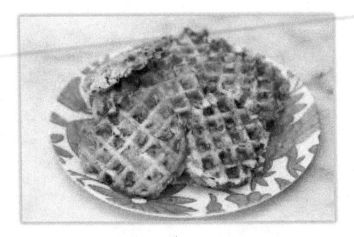

5 minutes

7 minutes

4 Servings

INGREDIENTS

½ cup of zucchini, grated

4 tablespoons of cream cheese, soft

1 tablespoon of almond

1 flour spoon of almonds, chopped

3 Eggs, beaten

1 tablespoon of steering

½ teaspoon of vanilla extract

DIRECTIONS

1. In a bowl, mix the zucchini with the cream cheese, almond flour and the other ingredients and blend well.

2. Heat the waffle iron over high heat, pour in ¼ of the batter, close the waffle maker, cook for 7 minutes and transfer to a plate.

3. Repeat with the remaining batter and serve the chaffles hot.

CURRY CHAFFLE

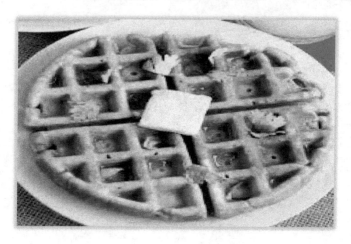

5 minutes

8 minutes

2 Servings

INGREDIENTS

1 egg, beaten

½ cup shredded mozzarella cheese

½ tsp curry powder

½ tsp fresh basil, finely chopped

DIRECTIONS

1. Heat up the waffle maker.

2. Add egg, shredded mozzarella cheese, curry powder and basil to a small mixing bowl and combine well.

3. Pour half of the batter into the waffle maker and cook for 4 minutes until brown. Repeat with the rest of the batter to make another chaffle.

4. Serve and enjoy!

SIMPLE CHAFFLE TOAST

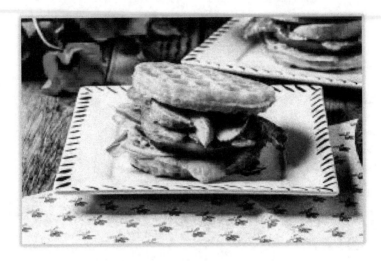

6 minutes

5 minutes

2 Servings

INGREDIENTS

1 large egg

1/2 cup shredded cheddar cheese

Toppings:

1 egg

3-4 spinach leaves

¼ cup boil and shredded chicken

DIRECTIONS

1. Preheat your square waffle maker on medium-high heat.

2. Mix together egg and cheese in a bowl and make two chaffles in a chaffle maker.

3. Once chaffle are cooked, carefully remove them from the maker.

4. Serve with spinach, boiled chicken, and fried egg.

5. Serve hot and enjoy!

SWISS CHEESE CHAFFLE

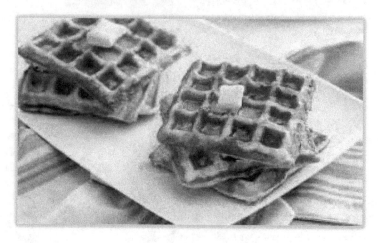

5 minutes

8 minutes

2 Servings

INGREDIENTS

1 large egg, beaten

½ cup of Swiss cheese, shredded

1 tbsp almond flour

DIRECTIONS

1. Heat up your waffle maker.

2. Add the cheese, almond flour, and egg to a tiny mixing bowl and combine well.

3. Pour half of the batter into your waffle maker and cook for 4 minutes until golden brown. Repeat now with the rest of the batter to make another chaffle.

4. Let cool for 3 minutes to let chaffles get crispy.

5. Serve and enjoy!

EASY SOFT CINNAMON ROLLS CHAFFLE CAKE

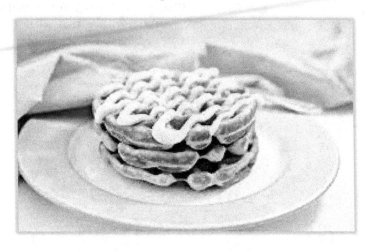

10 minutes

8 minutes

3Servings

INGREDIENTS

1 egg

1/2 cup mozzarella cheese

1/2 tsp. vanilla

1/2 tsp. cinnamon

1 tbs. monk fruit confectioner's blend

DIRECTIONS

1. Put the eggs in a small bowl. Add the remaining ingredients.

2. Spray to the chaffle maker with a non-stick cooking spray. Make two chaffles. Separate the mixture.

3. Cook half of the mixture for about 4 minutes or until golden. Notes Added Glaze: 1 tb. of cream cheese melted in a microwave for 15 seconds, and 1 tb. of monk fruit confectioners mix. Mix it and spread it over the moist fabric.

4. Additional Frosting: 1 tb. cream cheese (high temp), 1 tb room temp butter (low temp) and 1 tb monk fruit confectioners' mix.

5. Mix all the ingredients together and spread to the top of the cloth. Top with optional frosting, glaze, nuts, sugar-free syrup, whipped cream or simply dust with monk fruit sweets.

RICE KRISPIE TREAT CHAFFLE

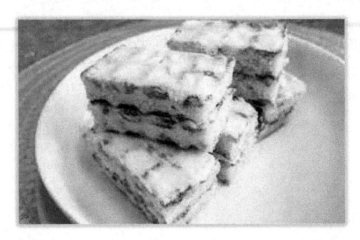

5 minutes

8 minutes

2 Servings

INGREDIENTS

Chaffle batter:

1 Egg

2-ounce Cream Cheese – softened

1/4 teaspoon Pure Vanilla Extract

2 tablespoons Lakanto Confectioners Sweetener

1-ounce Pork Rinds – crushed One teaspoon Baking Powder

Marshmallow Frosting:

DIRECTIONS

1. Preheat the waffle maker.

2. Add vanilla, egg, cream, and cheese into the mixing bowl and whisk until combine well.

3. Add baking powder, crushed pork rinds, and sweetener. Combine well until incorporated.

4. **Optional:** sprinkle crushed pork rinds onto the waffle maker.

5. After that, add ¼ of the batter into the waffle maker. Again, sprinkle pork rinds over the batter.

6. Let cook for three to four minutes and then let cool it. Repeat with the remaining batter.

1/4 cup Heavy Whipping Cream

1/4 teaspoon Pure Vanilla Extract

1 tablespoon Lakanto Confectioners Sweetener 1 teaspoon Xanthan Gum

7. Meanwhile, prepare the marshmallow frosting:

8. Whip the heavy whipping cream, confectioner, and vanilla until fluffy.

9. Sprinkle with xanthan gum and fold until incorporated.

10. Next, scatter frosting over chaffles and place into the fridge until set. Serve and enjoy!

CHOCOLATE CHIP CANNOLI CHAFFLE

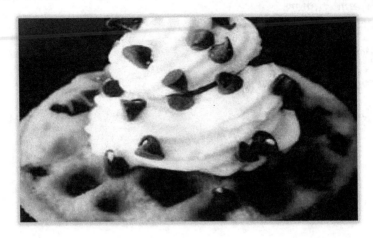

10 minutes

15 minutes

3 Servings

INGREDIENTS

Chocolate Chip Chaffle:

1 T Butter melted

1 T Golden Monkfruit sweetener

1 Egg Yolk

1/8 tsp Vanilla Extract

3 T Almond Flour

1/8 tsp Baking Powder

1 T Chocolate Chips sugar free

Cannoli Topping ingredients:

DIRECTIONS

1. Preheat the mini waffle maker.

2. In a small bowl, mix together all of the chaffle ingredients.

3. Place half of the ingredients in the mini waffle maker.

4. Cook the chaffle for about 3 to 4 minutes.

5. While the chaffle is cooking start making the Cannoli topping.

6. Add all of the ingredients for the Cannoli topping in a blender and blend everything together until it's smooth and creamy.

2oz Cream Cheese

*2 T Confectioners
Sweetener Low Carb*

6 T Ricotta full fat

1/4 tsp Vanilla Extract

5 drops Lemon Extract

CHOCOLATE CHERRY CHAFFLES

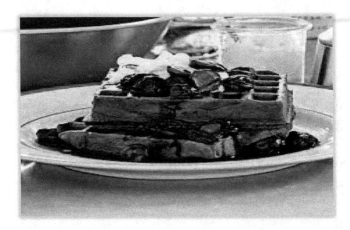

5 minutes

5 minutes

1 Servings

INGREDIENTS

1 Tbsp almond flour

1 Tbsp cocoa powder

1Tbsp sugar free sweetener

½ tsp baking powder

1 whole egg

½ cup mozzarella cheese shredded

2 Tbsp heavy whipping cream whipped

2 Tbsp sugar free cherry pie filling

1 Tbsp chocolate chips

DIRECTIONS

1. Turn on waffle maker to heat and oil it with cooking spray.

2. Mix all dry components in a bowl.

3. Add egg and mix well.

4. Add cheese and stir again.

5. Spoon batter into waffle maker and close.

6. Cook for 5 minutes, until done.

7. Top with whipping cream, cherries, and chocolate chips.

HERB PIZZA CHAFFLE

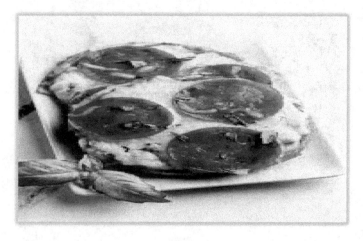

5minutes

8minutes

2 Servings

INGREDIENTS

2 egg, beaten

½ teaspoon of dried oregano

½ teaspoon of dried basil

½ teaspoon of parsley flakes

½ teaspoon of garlic powder

1spoons of tomato sauce

1 cup shredded mozzarella, shredded

DIRECTIONS

1. In a bowl, mix the egg with the aromatic herbs and half of the mozzarella and mix well.

2. Preheat the waffle iron over medium-high heat, pour in half the chaffle mixture, cook for 4 minutes and transfer to a plate.

3. Repeat with the rest of the batter, spread the tomato puree and the rest of the cheese on the chaffles and serve.

PECANS CHAFFLE

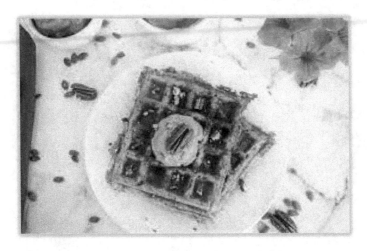

5 minutes

8 minutes

2 Servings

INGREDIENTS

1 tbsp almond flour

½ cup mozzarella cheese 1 egg, beaten

1 tbsp sweetener

½ tsp vanilla extract

For topping:

1 tbsp whipped cream

1 tbsp unsweetened maple syrup

½ cup of chopped pecans

DIRECTIONS

1. Heat up the waffle maker.

2. Pour ½ of the batter into your waffle maker and cook for 4 minutes. Then cook the remaining batter to make another chaffle.

3. Top the chaffles with keto whipped cream, maple syrup and sprinkle with chopped pecans.

4. Serve and enjoy!

ROSEMARY CHAFFLES

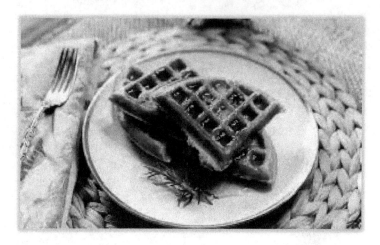

5 minutes

5 minutes

2 Servings

INGREDIENTS

1 organic egg, beaten

1/2 cup Cheddar cheese, shredded

1 tbspn almond flour

1 tbspn fresh rosemary, chopped

DIRECTIONS

1. Preheat now a mini waffle iron and then grease it.

2. In a bowl, place all ingredients and with a fork, Mix well until well combined.

3. Place half of the mixture into Preheat nowed waffle iron and cook for about 4 minutes or until golden brown.

4. Repeat now with the remaining mixture.

FLAXSEED CHAFFLE

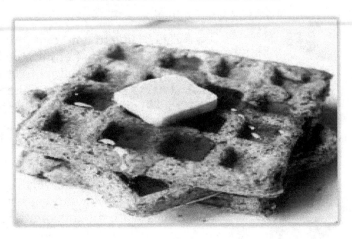

10 minutes

20 minutes

4 Servings

INGREDIENTS

2 cups ground flaxseed

2 teaspoons ground cinnamon

1 teaspoon of sea salt

1 tablespoon baking powder

1/3 cup / 80 ml avocado oil

5 eggs, at room temperature

½ cup / 120 ml water

Whipped cream as needed for topping

DIRECTIONS

1. Take a non-stick waffle iron, plug it in, select the medium or medium-high heat setting and let it preheat until ready to use; it could also be indicated with an indicator light changing its color.

2. Meanwhile, the batter and for this, take a large bowl and then stir in flaxseed, salt and baking powder until combined.

3. Crack the eggs in a jug, pour in oil and water, whisk these ingredients until blended and then stir this mixture into the flour with the spatula until incorporated and fluffy mixture comes together.

4. Let the batter stand for 5 minutes and then stir in cinnamon until mixed.

5. Use a ladle to pour one-fourth of the prepared batter into the heated waffle iron in a spiral direction, starting from the edges, then shut the lid and cooking for 5 minutes or more until solid and nicely browned; the cooked waffle will look like a cake.

6. When done, transfer chaffle to a plate with a silicone spatula and repeat with the remaining batter.

7. Top waffles with whipped cream and then serve straight away.

KETO PEANUT BUTTER CHAFFLE CAKE

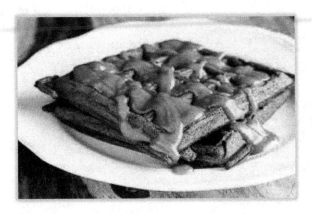

8 minutes

10 minutes

2 Servings

INGREDIENTS

For peanut butter chaffle:

2 Tbs. Sugar-Free Peanut Butter Powder

2 Tbs. Monkfruit Confectioner's

1 egg

1/4 teaspoon baking powder

1 Tbs. Heavy Whipped Cream

1/4 teaspoon peanut butter extract

Peanut butter frosting:

DIRECTIONS

1. Put the eggs in a small bowl. Add the ingredients and mix well until the dough is smooth and creamy.

2. If you don't have peanut butter extract, you can skip it.

3. It adds absolutely wonderful, more powerful peanut butter flavor and is worth investing in this extract.

4. Pour half of the butter into a mini chaffle maker and cook for 2-3 minutes until it is completely cooked. In another small bowl, add sweetener, cream cheese, sugar-free natural peanut butter and vanilla.

5. Mix frosting until everything is well blended. When the chaffle cake has completely cooled to room temperature, spread on the

55

2 Tbs. Monkfruit
Confectioners

1 Tbs. butter softens,
room temperature

1 tbs. unsweetened
natural peanut butter
or peanut butter
powder

2 Tbs. cream cheese
softens, room
temperature

1/4 tsp. vanilla

frosting. Or you can even pipe on the frosting! Or you can heat the frosting and add 1/2 teaspoon of water to make the peanut butter glaze and drizzle over the peanut butter chaffle!

ALMOND JOY CAKE CHAFFLE

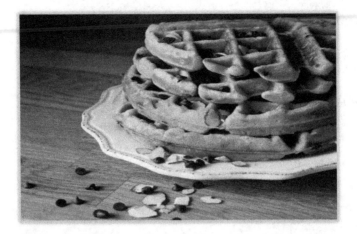

5minutes

10 minutes

2 Servings

INGREDIENTS

1 egg

1-ounce cream cheese

1 tablespoon almond flour

1 tablespoon unsweetened cocoa powder

1 tablespoon erythritol sweetener blend such as Swerve, Pyure or Lakanto

½ teaspoon vanilla extract

1/4 teaspoon instant coffee powder

DIRECTIONS

1. Preheat the waffle iron.

2. Whisk all chaffle ingredients into the bowl until mixed well. Add half of the batter into the preheated waffle iron.

3. Cook for three to five minutes.

4. When done, remove and let cool them. Repeat with 2nd chaffle.

For the Filling:

1. Soften cream in the microwave oven for ten seconds or room temperature.

2. Add all ingredients into a medium bowl and combine well until smooth.

Coconut filling:

1 1/2 teaspoons coconut oil melted

1 tablespoon heavy cream

1/4 cup unsweetened finely shredded coconut

2 ounce cream cheese

1 tablespoon confectioners sweetener such as Swerve

1/4 teaspoon vanilla extract

14 whole almonds

3. Next, scatter half of the filling on the chaffle and put seven almonds over the filling.

4. Repeat with 2nd chaffle.

KETO CAULIFLOWER CHAFFLES

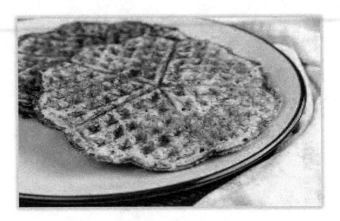

5 minutes

4 minutes

2 Servings

INGREDIENTS

1 cup riced cauliflower

1/4 teaspoon Garlic Powder

1/4 teaspoon Ground Black Pepper

1/2 teaspoon Italian Seasoning

1/4 teaspoon Salt

1/2 cup shredded mozzarella cheese or shredded mexican blend cheese

1 egg

1/2 cup shredded parmesan cheese

DIRECTIONS

1. Add all ingredients into a blender.

2. Sprinkle 1/8 cup parmesan cheese into the waffle maker. Make sure to cover the bottom of the waffle iron.

3. Fill the waffle maker with the cauliflower mixture.

4. Add another sprinkle of parmesan cheese on top of the mixture.

5. Cook for 4-5 minutes, or until crispy.

6. Makes 4 mini chaffles, or two regular full-size chaffles.

OREO COOKIE CHAFFLE

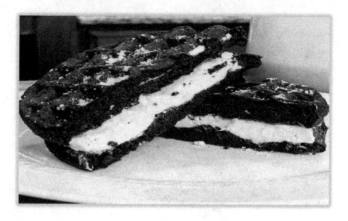

5 minutes

10 minutes

3 Servings

INGREDIENTS

1 egg

1 tbs black cocoa

1 tbs monkfruit confectioners blend or your favorite keto-approved sweetener

1/4 tsp baking powder

2 tbs cream cheese room temperature and softened

1 tbs mayonnaise

1/4 tsp instant coffee powder not liquid

pinch salt

DIRECTIONS

1. In a small bowl, whip up the egg.

2. Add the remaining ingredients and mix well until the batter is smooth and creamy.

3. Divide the batter into 3 and pour each in a mini waffle maker and cook it for 2 1/2 to 3 minutes until it's fully cooked.

4. In a separate small bowl, add the sweetener, cream cheese, and vanilla. Mix the frosting until everything is well incorporated.

5. Spread the frosting on the waffle cake after it has completely cooled down to room temperature.

1 tsp vanilla

**Frosting
ingredients:**

*2 Tbs monkfruit
confectioners*

*2 Tbs cream cheese
softened and room
temp*

1/4 tsp clear vanilla

CHURRO WAFFLES

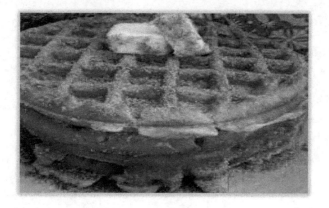

5 minutes

10 minutes

1Servings

INGREDIENTS

1 tbsp coconut cream

1 egg

6 tbsp almond flour

¼ tsp xanthan gum

½ tsp cinnamon

2 tbsp keto brown sugar

Coating:

2 tbsp butter, melt

1 tbsp keto brown sugar Warm up your waffle maker.

DIRECTIONS

1. Pour half of the batter to the waffle pan and cook for 5 minutes.

2. Carefully remove the cooked waffle and repeat the steps with the remaining batter.

3. Allow the chaffles to cool and spread with the melted butter and top with the brown sugar.

MUSHROOM CHAFFLE

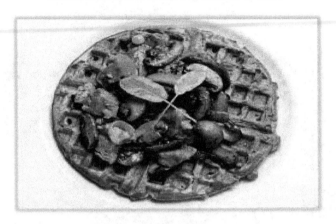

5 minutes

6 minutes

2 Servings

INGREDIENTS

2 beaten eggs

½ cup of mozzarella, chopped

½ cup of mushrooms, sliced teaspoon of coriander, ground

½ teaspoon of dried rosemary

½ teaspoon of cayenne pepper spoons of tomato sauce

DIRECTIONS

1. In a bowl, mix the eggs with the mozzarella, coriander, rosemary, and cayenne pepper and mix well.

2. Preheat the waffle iron over medium-high heat, pour half the chaffle mixture, cook for 6 minutes and transfer to a plate.

3. Repeat with the rest of the batter, spread the puree and mushrooms on the chaffles and serve.

PEANUT BUTTER AND STRAWBERRY JAM CHAFFLE

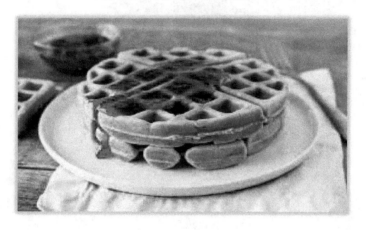

10 minutes

14 minutes

2 Servings

INGREDIENTS

2 eggs, beaten

2 tbsp almond flour

½ tsp baking powder

1 tbsp strawberry jam, sugar-free

2 tbsp peanut butter

1 cup mozzarella cheese, shredded

1 tbsp cream cheese

DIRECTIONS

1. Heat up the waffle maker.

2. Add all the chaffles ingredients to a small mixing bowl and stir until well combined.

3. Pour 1/6 of the batter into the waffle maker and cook for 4 minutes until brown. Repeat with the rest of the batter to prepare the other chaffles.

4. Let cool for 2-3 minutes to let chaffles get crispy.

5. Serve and enjoy!

CRUNCH CEREAL CAKE CHAFFLE

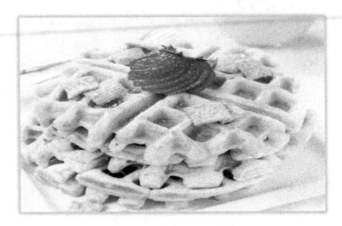

10 minutes

5 minutes

1 Servings

INGREDIENTS

1 egg

2 tbsp. almond flour

1/2 tsp. coconut flour

1 tbsp. butter, melted

1 tbsp. cream cheese, softened

1/4 tsp. vanilla extract

1/4 tsp. baking powder

1 tbsp. confectioners' sweetener

1/8 tsp. xanthan gum

For the toppings:

DIRECTIONS

1. Preheat the mini waffle maker.

2. Blend or mix all the chaffles ingredients until the consistency is creamy and smooth. Allow to rest for a few minutes so that the flour absorbs the liquid ingredients.

3. Scoop out 2-3 tbsp. of batter and put it into the waffle maker. Allow to cooking for 2-3 minutes.

4. Top the cooked chaffles with freshly whipped cream.

5. Add syrup and drops of Captain Cereal flavoring for a great flavor.

*20 drops captain
cereal flavoring*

Whipped cream

UBE CHAFFLES WITH ICE CREAM

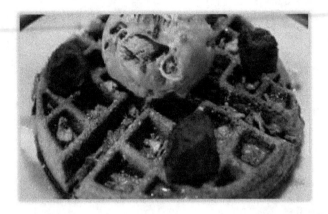

5 minutes

10 minutes

2 Servings

INGREDIENTS

1/3 cup mozzarella cheese, shredded

1 tbsp whipped cream cheese

2 tbsp sweetener

1 egg

2-3 drops ube or pandan extract

1/2 tsp baking powder

Keto ice cream

DIRECTIONS

1. Add in 2 or 3 drops of ube extract, mix until creamy and smooth.

2. Pour half of the batter mixture in the mini waffle maker and cook for about 5 minutes.

3. Repeat the same steps with the remaining batter mixture.

4. Top with keto ice cream and enjoy.

KETO RYE BREAD CHAFFLE

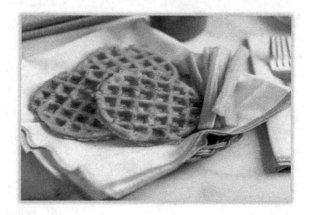

10 minutes

20 minutes

2 Servings

INGREDIENTS

1 egg

2 tbsps almond flour

1 tbspn Melt nowed butter

1 tbspn mozzarella cheese

pinch salt

pinch garlic powder

1/2 teaspoon baking powder

1/2 teaspoon caraway seeds

DIRECTIONS

1. Preheat now mini waffle maker.

2. Mix all rye bread chaffle ingredients in a tiny bowl.

3. Place 1/2 the mixture into a Preheat nowed mini waffle maker.

4. Cook for 4 minutes.

5. Serve warm.

NUTMEG CHAFFLE

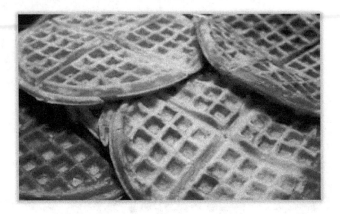

5 minutes

5 minutes

2 Servings

INGREDIENTS

3 tablespoons of cream

1 tablespoon of coconut oil, melted

1 tablespoon of coconut flour

1 egg, beaten spoonful of stevia

½ teaspoon of ground nutmeg spoons of cream cheese

½ teaspoon of vanilla extract

DIRECTIONS

1. In a bowl, mix the cream with the coconut oil, egg and other ingredients and beat well.

2. Heat the waffle iron over high heat, pour half the batter in, close the waffle maker, cook for 5 minutes and transfer to a plate.

3. Repeat with the remaining batter and serve.

KETO BOSTON CREAM PIE CHAFFLE CAKE

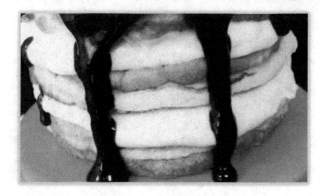

10 minutes

10 minutes

4 Servings

INGREDIENTS

2 eggs

1/4 cup almond flour
Coconut flour

1 teaspoon

2 tablespoons of
melted butter

2 tablespoons of cream
cheese

20 drops of Boston
Cream Extract

1/2 teaspoon of vanilla
extract

1/2 teaspoon baking
powder

DIRECTIONS

1. Preheat the mini chaffle iron to render the cake chops first.

2. Mix all the ingredients of the cake and blend until smooth and fluffy. It's only supposed to take a few minutes. Heat the heavy whipping cream to a boil on the stovetop. When it's dry, whisk the egg yolks together in a small separate dish.

3. Once the cream is boiling, add half of it to the egg yolks. Make sure you're whisking it together while you're slowly pouring it into the mixture. Take off from the heat and whisk in your vanilla and xanthan gum. Then set aside to cool and thicken.

4. Place the ganache ingredients in a small bowl. Microwave for about

2 tablespoons sweetener or monk fruit

1/4 teaspoon xanthan powder

Custard Ingredients:

1/2 cup fresh cream

1/2 teaspoon of vanilla extract

1/2 tbs. Swerve confectioners Sweetener

2 egg yolks

1/8 teaspoon xanthan gum

Ingredients for ganache:

2 tbs. heavy whipped cream

2 tbs. unsweetened baking chocolate bar chopped

1 tbs. Swerve Confectioners sweetener

20 seconds, stir. Repeat, if necessary.

5. Be careful not to overheat and roast the ganache.

6. Just do it 20 seconds at a time until it's completely melted. Assemble and enjoy your Boston Cream Pie Chaffle Cake!!

APPLE PIE CHURRO CHAFFLE TACOS

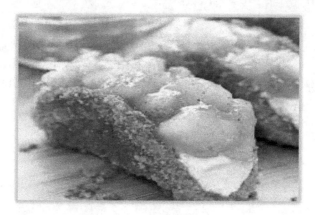

10 minutes

30 minutes

4 Servings

INGREDIENTS

1 Chayote Squash cooked – peeled and sliced

1 tablespoon butter

2 packages True Lemon

1/8 teaspoon cream of tartar

1/4 cup Swerve Brown

2 teaspoons cinnamon powder

1/8 teaspoon ginger powder

1/8 teaspoon nutmeg

DIRECTIONS

Apple pie taco filling:

1. First, boil the whole chayote for twenty-five minutes. Cool it. Peel and cut into the ¼-inch slice.

2. Combine all ingredients and add chayote to cover well.

3. Put on the baking sheet, cover it with foil and bake for twenty minutes.

4. Add ¼ mixtures into the blender and process until you get a sauce consistency. Add to chayote slices and stir well.

Apple pie churro chaffle taco:

1. First, whip the eggs. Add vanilla, cinnamon, and sweetener to the whipped egg and combine well.

Cinnamon Chaffle:

2 eggs

1/4 cup mozzarella – shredded

1 teaspoon cinnamon

1 tablespoon Swerve Confectioners

2 teaspoons coconut flour

1/8 tsp baking powder

1 teaspoon vanilla extract

2. Next, add the remaining ingredients and combine well. Add three tablespoons of batter into the waffle maker.

3. Let cook for five minutes. Sprinkle with granulated sweetener and cinnamon.

4. Place chaffles in taco holders or fold them. Add ¼ of apple filling into each taco chaffle.